LOSE YOUR THIGHS!
and your legs will fall off

by Rebecca Parks Barnard

Inventor of the LimbaSlim® Weight Release System

Lose Your Thighs! and your legs will fall off

Copyright ©2009 Rebecca Parks Barnard

All rights reserved

Cover design by Rebecca

adapted from William Bouguereau, *The Wave*, 1896

Pen and ink illustrations by Bryn Barnard

ISBN: 978-0-557-05356-8

For permission, contact

Limba Systems, LLC

417 Point Caution Drive

Friday Harbor, WA 98250

Rebecca@LimbaSystems.com

Printed in the United States

TABLE OF CONTENTS

Introduction   5

Chapter 1   LOOK AT ME. NO, DON'T.   13

Chapter 2   YOU'RE GETTING SLEEEEEEEEPY   19

Chapter 3   GREAT AUNT HANNAH   25

Chapter 4   JULIE DONUT   33

Chapter 5   DON'T TORTURE YOURSELF   39

A Little Test   43

Chapter 6   DESIRE   47

Chapter 7   CHEATING   55

Chapter 8   YOUR GROOVY BRAIN   61

Chapter 9   THE LIMBIC SYSTEM   65

Chapter 10 EATING CLOSE TO THE EARTH   71

The List   73

A Sample Daily Menu   83

Chapter 11 THE FIRST DAY   89

Chapter 12 PLEASE DON'T EAT THE POODLES   93

Recipes   101

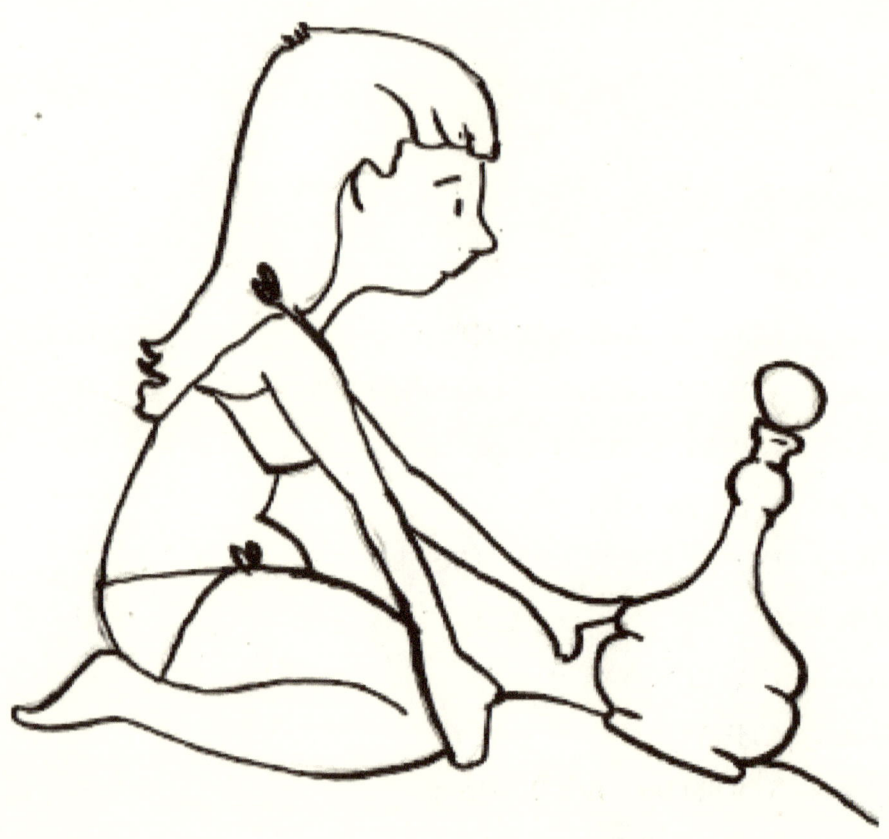

INTRODUCTION

If you found a genie in a bottle and had three wishes,
would at least one of them have to do with
getting thinner?

I am a regular woman. A proud mother. An artsy hausfrau. A business owner, inventor, writer, dreamer.   And for many years, every time I passed a mirror, all I could see was my thighs.

Men don't think like this. If they look in a mirror at all, they just suck in their guts and walk on by.   If we've come such a long way, baby, why are 21st century women still in the 1950s when it comes to self image?

I hope you bought this book because you are ready to take your body back and allow it to be as healthy as can be. But if you think you will have to suffer for this to happen, think again.

Eating is a wonderful thing. Our appetites are a gift, and fighting them is just plain silly. In these pages, you will learn to love your body, to feed it right, and to retrain your habits - because once we make peace with our bodies and our appetites – and add in a trick or two – we will be on the road to our perfect weight FOREVER.

My goal in writing this book is to empower all women,
so that when we do find that genie in the bottle,
we really will all wish – three times – for world peace.

It's worth a shot.

BEFORE WE START, DO THIS

Please fill out this little self assessment. Go ahead, write in the book. Unless it's from the library.

1. MY NAME is:

_____

2. If I could be anything on this list,

I would most wish to be:

      a. faster

      b. slimmer

      c. healthier

      d. happier

      e. smarter

3. Of the following, I can get most excited about:

   a. a perfectly ripe peach

   b. beans, tortillas and salsa

   c. a big green salad with vinaigrette

   d. a hot bowl of creamy potato soup

Next, use your answers from the questions above to fill in the blanks in the following sentence:

I, _____ (answer from 1)

feel _____(answer from 2)

when I eat _____(answer from 3)

NOW: Write your sentence ten times, either here or on a separate paper.

Say it out loud. Yell it. Whisper it.
Do this every day until you get bored with it.

THE CONTRACT

I,

_____/

hereby vow to read <u>Lose Your Thighs</u> with an open mind and heart.

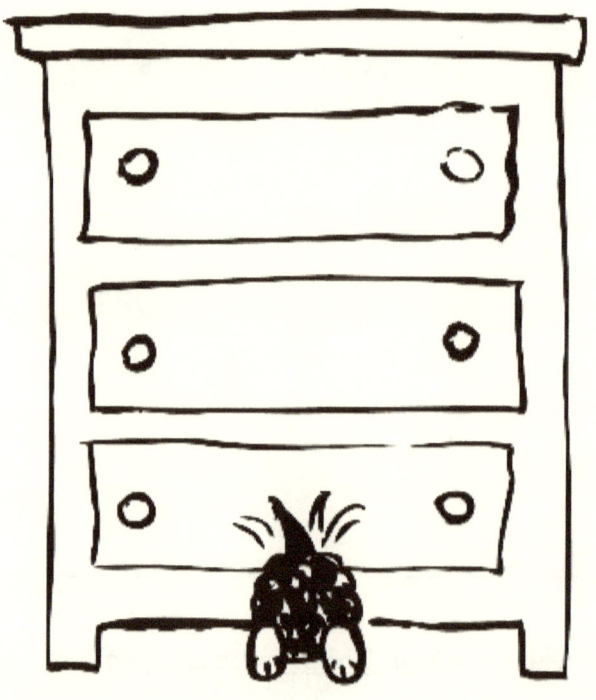

1

Look At Me. No, Don't.

When I was a child, we had a dog named Scott, whom we loved tremendously even though he kept biting us.   The biting wasn't Scott's only endearing trait. He really was cute, in that ugly kind of way. His crooked teeth, his bad breath, bow legs, terrible personality...we couldn't imagine life without Scott.

There was one thing that Scott did that my family thought was particularly clever. When he wanted us not to find him, he would hide his head under a dresser. Just his head. His whole body would be visible, in fact if you said his name, his tail would wag, but Scott was certain he couldn't be seen. We loved that about Scott. He was a real dog's dog.

I bring this up because I have recently learned something that reminds me of Scott.

Do you have a body part you want to hide? A part you feel sure is uglier, fatter, bonier, jigglier, more spotted than anyone else's? A part that dictates every piece of clothing you buy? Come on. I know you do. Every woman does – at least every woman who feels overweight, and I can assume you bought this book because you feel you are overweight.

You probably also have a part that you love. Sure you do. Maybe it's your nose. Your boobs. Your neck or shoulders. Your back. Your eyebrows. Your teeth or your toes. Something you appreciate.

So here's the question: Which part do you look at first when you face a mirror?

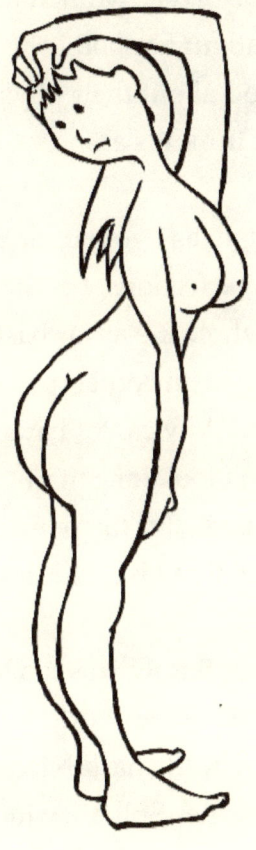

For most of us, it's the "Bad Part."

Given enough time, probably every woman in the U.S. – even thin ones - can find something about her body she hates. Even those women who feel pretty good about their physical selves will find a flaw that looms huge in their minds alone.

One day not long ago enough, as I got out of the shower and did the quick full body scan for imperfections, I realized how much this sucks. EVERY day of my whole life as far back as I can remember, I have looked at my reflection with contempt. Those legs. NO one has legs like mine. My big butt. Why can't I have a little bikini butt like my friend so and so? I didn't look long at my amazingly good parts - and there were some of course. But the point isn't that I didn't look at the Good Parts. The point is that I labeled the others Bad.

I was a child in the 1960s. My family was too late to be hippies, though they professed liberal - even World Federalist - ideology, protested the Vietnam War and Richard Nixon, and consistently voted for civil and female rights. Still, they judged every woman they saw by her looks. I remember my father saying that he didn't understand the fuss about the beauty of Jackie Kennedy - because "her thighs don't meet at the top." I never really got this comment (still don't) but I didn't know enough then even to disagree with the notion that the *First Lady* - a fine and intelligent woman - was judged as less than worthy because of *the shape of the tops of her legs*.

I never heard my parents say anything about men's looks. Nada. Just the women. Eleanor Roosevelt? Well, we all know about her little ugliness problem. What a shame. She could have achieved so much.

Sheesh.

It makes me crazy still. And it bothers me that it took so many years to break this habit in myself - of looking critically at every (female) body. Those habitual paths were friggin' freeways in my brain that I blithely traveled without thinking for the next 10 years. Although it wasn't easy to change and took me many years, I am proud to report that those paths are off the map now.

So back to that day not so long ago when I got out of the shower: I had an epiphany. As I began my usual assessment - GOD your legs are **huge** – must buy baggier pants - I stopped myself. I turned away. I averted my eyes from my thighs and made a decision NOT to look at my legs that day. Every time I passed a mirror, I could look at any other part: My face. My arms. My hair. But not my legs. Or my butt.

And guess what happened. All day long I felt thinner. I felt fitter. I felt **normal**. Maybe it was my crone's wisdom kicking in as I approached menopause. Whatever it was, I continue to be grateful for that morning.

 I no longer look only at my flaws. It took some training, but now it is second nature.

Try it.

Lest you think this is yet another "Blame the victim" dealio, I remind you that this self-loathing *isn't our fault*. We live in a media-saturated world. Our thoughts are manipulated every day. Advertising shapes our will, our diet, our habits. Fat-free models on magazine covers whittle away our inherent belief in the gorgeous perfection of the curvy female. Advertisers stuff us with insecurity because it is a powerful selling tool: **Make a woman feel less-than**, and she will be primed to buy a product that promises improvement.

"Oooh, if I use that [lotion, makeup, diet, chemical] I'll look like that model. If I don't, well, it's my own fault that I'm such a lump." The standard is impossible. So it keeps us buying.

Even if we don't watch TV, we can't escape the body-impossible media images all around us. Our minds are beautifully compliant - when our brain receives a suggestion, it does its best to follow it. Self-fulfilling prophecy is a well-known factor in parent-child counseling:

Tell a child she's clumsy, and she will become so.

Tell a woman she's fat - and her body will try its best to comply.

Although this is a fact I can't verify,

I am fairly certain cave women didn't do this.

18

2

You're Getting Sleeeeeeeeepy

Walk up to someone who is fully aware, totally "present", and tell them you can program their mind to make them quack like a duck whenever they hear the word "pickle." Go ahead, try it.

Okay, I know you won't really do that - because you know it won't work, and the person would think you were nuts. "I will not," they'd say. And they're right: they probably wouldn't - because their conscious brain is smarter than that. Freud called it the ego – the part of the mind that censors data. A fully awake human being is largely protected by this gatekeeper – keeping out unnecessary data and allowing only the self-benefiting stuff to enter and stay.

Stage hypnotists know that in order to "program" someone, her conscious mind and its barriers must first be disarmed. So before they plant any suggestions (like "you will quack like a duck,") they must first change the victim's brain state so that her mind is wide open. It isn't difficult, given a few tricks. It's basically just guidance into a deep relaxation, where the censoring mind is off-duty.

BETA, ALPHA, THETA, DELTA[1]

There are four main brainwave states. Each of us goes in and out of these states many times daily, and in a nice tidy order whenever we fall asleep. The different states can be tracked in brain scanning machinery. I am not a neuroscientist, but the basics are this:

In a totally awake, conscious state, you are in the Beta brainwave state. Whenever you are fully aware, concentrating, such as when you are immersed in a conversation, your brainwaves are their quickest, and you are "in Beta."

Many times during the day, our minds wander into one of the *subconscious* states, the lightest of which is Alpha. The frequency of our brainwaves slows down, and we are less aware, but still totally awake. This is the state of light meditation. When you take a walk alone, you are probably in Alpha. Alpha feels good. It's a bit

---

[1] Yes, the order is not right, according to the Greek alphabet. I suspect some early researcher goofed up, and we're left with Beta, Alpha, Theta, Delta. I tried to fix it, but those snooty neuroscientists haven't returned my calls.

detached from reality, but still functioning. Kids live mostly in Alpha. It's the "eyes-glazed-over, lost in thought" feeling. My mother used to call this state, "gathering wool." As in, "You can't talk to him, he's gathering wool."

The next subconscious state is that delicious state of devoted daydreaming, called Theta. Have you ever found yourself 10 miles down the freeway en route somewhere, and don't remember a thing about the road you've just traveled? You might say your "mind was somewhere else." That's a light form of Theta. At a deeper level, Theta is a light sleep. Not unconscious, but subconscious - the Powernap state. Some of our best ideas come to us while we are in the Theta brainwave state. It is the favorite of hypnotists, and is the state we are most interested in here.[2] It is during Theta that the ego is shut off, and our brains work most freely, unencumbered by guilt or censorship. Theta is also the state during which the mind is most suggestible; the conscious Beta monitor is on a break.

And whaddya know. When we watch TV or a movie, guess at the frequency of our brainwaves. Yup. Alpha and Theta. It's brilliant. This means we are wide open for suggestion, a fact of which advertisers are well aware.

---

[2] The fourth state is Delta, or deep sleep. Within Delta, there is actually a state where you are so totally unconscious that someone could cut you and you wouldn't feel it. But that's further than we need to go today.

While the gatekeeper is distracted, the commercial programming goes in without censorship or resistance. We are sure - with every fiber of our raveling self-esteem - that we aren't valuable unless our thighs are the same diameter as Jennifer Aniston's, yet we are also absolutely sure that we need that 10-cheese pizza, right now.

This is where we fight back. Yes, advertisers can stuff impossible self-esteem-bashing notions into our brains.
But no one can make us quack like a duck unless we let them. They are **our** brains. And ultimately we alone control them.

In the 1970s, in a quixotic quest to heal my childhood-shattered self, I took some classes in self-hypnosis. All hypnosis works on the principle of suggestibility: implanting a suggestion when the brain is in a super-relaxed and receptive brainwave state (which we now know is called Theta.) During a hypnosis session, the hypnotist relaxes the patient through a prescribed series of steps. First the body is relaxed, and gradually the mind follows. Once the hypnotist can see that the patient's brainwaves have sufficiently slowed, she begins with the suggestions: "You are thin. You are a healthy non-smoker. You pass the bar exam with the highest score ever recorded." Whatever the goal, after the session, the patients walks out of the office feeling invulnerable, strong, chockfull of emotional wellbeing and strength.

Hypnosis can be very effective. For a while. But soon the calm of the hypnotic suggestions wears thin and has to be repeated. This is why I studied self-hypnosis – there was no way I could afford hundred-dollar weekly sessions with a real hypnotherapist. I was looking for something permanent that I could do myself.

It worked, kind of. But I grew bored with it, and it became impossible to imagine doing this self-hypnosis thing for the rest of my life. I knew I needed to find a better – easier - way to get inside my brain and fix it. If hypnosis didn't do it, what was left?

Drugs? No way. They make us sick and might kill us.

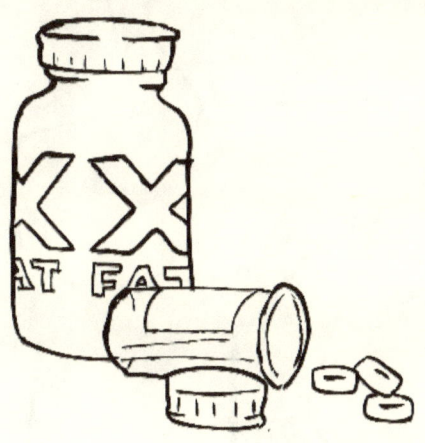

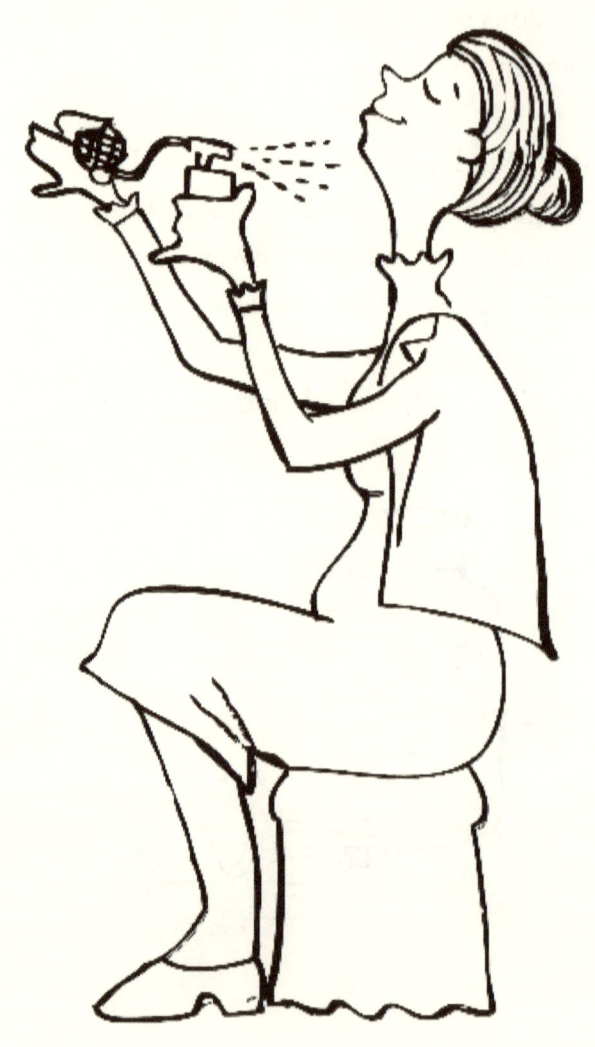

3

Great Aunt Hannah

Aunt Hannah was 75 years old when I was born, but I remember her driving my brothers and me around town in her big blue 1953 Oldsmobile Rocket. We figured she dyed her hair to match that car. Aunt Hannah was from that old school of ladies who wore gloves and hats. And she always smelled SO good.

Years later, long after Hannah was gone, I was at a meeting and noticed an oddly familiar fragrance. Someone was wearing Hannah's perfume, and the memory immediately transported me back to that big blue car, Hannah at the wheel in her hat and gloves. It felt as if I was there - not dreaming it, not thinking about it - but THERE.

I began to realize how smells have that ability - to transport us, to trigger memories long forgotten. The smell of the ocean on a particular day, the smell of a certain flower in bloom - out of the blue, a long-forgotten sniff can take us back in time. We all have experienced this. Science calls it olfactory memory.[3]

It occurred to me that if the smell of Aunt Hannah's perfume in a meeting could produce such a vivid memory experience, and transport me so totally into another dimension, it must be triggering my brain to enter one of the slower brainwave states - without my even trying. It was a short leap to wonder if the mind might not be particularly open to suggestion in this situation.

In the 1990s, I had worked for a lavender farm and learned a bit about aromatherapy. I adored how lavender relaxed me, and shared this with the customers seeking to eliminate stress. It worked – sales were high and customers came back. But I noticed something else, even more profound. Every morning when I opened the store and released the day's wave of fragrance from of the luscious lavender bouquets that lined the walls, I was transported back to a beautiful summer vacation I had taken in France as a single woman, many years before. How I relished that feeling! When my co-workers saw me stop, close my eyes and take a deep breath, I imagine they assumed I was soaking up the calming fragrance of the lavender products all around me. They didn't know that I was mentally back in Nice in 1978, lying topless on a beach with *mon amour d'été*.

---

[3] More about the science in chapter 8

I knew I was on to something. Over the years, I had taken enough courses to call myself a hypnotist, although I hadn't practiced hypnosis on anyone outside my own family and myself. I decided to try something: I would combine a new hypnosis with a new fragrance, with the intention of creating a new, powerful olfactory memory that could be triggered later by simply smelling the same fragrance.

I wrote and recorded a 10-minute self-hypnosis that spoke to all the weight-related issues I knew to be ingrained in my head because of advertising and Hollywood. First, I guided the listener (me) through a series of relaxation exercises. Then we took a walk on a beautiful beach, as I spoke of respecting the gift of my appetite, of loving my body, and desiring only whole, healthful foods that honored it. I didn't mention being overweight, or weight loss. It was all positive – loving good food, loving my body, respecting my appetite.

Because it was already so familiar to me, I knew I needed to distance myself from the CD, which I did by not listening to it for a month after it was finished. When the day came to give it a try – and here's where Hannah comes in - *before I pressed Play, I took a deep whiff of a new fragrance.*

I listened to the meditation. It was lovely (if I do say so myself) – a complete beta-alpha-theta journey. When I finished listening, I was refreshed and strong, like after any hypnosis session.

But this time was different.

For the rest of that day, I carried the fragrance around with me, and *whenever I was tempted to overeat, I took a little sniff.*

It worked! The scent triggered my olfactory memory of the hypnosis! Immediately, my mind went back to the beautiful beach, and I was enveloped in a feeling of respect for my body and appetite. Just a sniff made me strong, and it lasted all day. I truly didn't want to eat anything except whole, healthful foods. I listened again the next day, and then every day for the first week. I always carried my little fragrance with me.

After a week, I began skipping sessions (because I am basically lazy – I mean busy) and just sniffed the fragrance. When I felt I was slipping back, I would listen again. I proceeded in this way – the intervals between listenings getting longer and longer, but always carrying the fragrance with me for strength – until eventually I didn't need to listen anymore at all. The olfactory memory was fully entrenched – I knew that forever after I would only need to sniff that particular scent to reactivate it.

My brain had changed. I had found a way in.

I did some more research about the power of specific scents, and eventually came up with the luscious mixture I called LimbaScent. It is a mix of grapefruit and a secret ingredient – all organic, of course. (I knew I had to be sure it was a unique fragrance to anyone who smelled if for the first time, so I added a tiny bit of a secret natural essential oil that gave LimbaScent its unique molecular profile.)

I made 20 copies of the meditation, and packed them with pocket-sized LimbaSniffers that I filled at my dining room table.

Then I offered it to anyone I could find whom I knew to be struggling with weight and body image issues. (This was practically every woman I knew.)

The reports began coming in. Here are three:

Dear Rebecca,

I just got my LimbaSlim package in the mail five days ago, and I have to tell you, I'm so glad I did. My urge to overeat, and especially to eat junk food, seems to have melted away.

Only one day after starting on LimbaSlim, I drove effortlessly past my worst temptation of the week: fresh cookies, lovingly hand made by a professional baker, and only sold once a week. I couldn't believe I was driving right by like that, and that it was so easy!

Thank you!

Christine

Anchorage, Alaska

Dear Rebecca,

What I love about the LimbaSlim program is how simple and easy it is. The meditation CD is less than 10 minutes long, so it's easy to fit into my schedule. No excuses. I find my eating habits are leaning towards healthier foods now; And when I am tempted by things I know I shouldn't eat, I get out my little Sniffer and take a couple deep whiffs of that lovely sweet grapefruit aroma. YUM! It really brings my mind back to the image of the healthy fit body I desire. My resolve is strengthened and I am making better choices.

I have already lost 6 pounds! And that is the very best part!

MaryAnn
Phoenix, AZ

Dear LimbaSlim

It's been months since your cd and aromatherapy inhaler arrived. I used it diligently for a few weeks. The inhaler is next to my computer and I still use it every morning.

On May 1st, my daughter and I walked from her house to a special little deli and I had my first encounter with raw foods. I was blown away by how delicious the food was. Since then, my entire food-related lifestyle has been gradually changing and improving.

On your cd, you describe the table on the beach laden with beautiful and delicious fresh, living food, and you draw the listener to the table and have her sample what is there. This morning, I realized that your guided visualization has manifested. My own table, on a smaller scale, looks like that more and more frequently lately. Oh, and I'm several pounds lighter after a long, dry spell. Thank you so much for your "magic wand."
Love,

Catherine
California

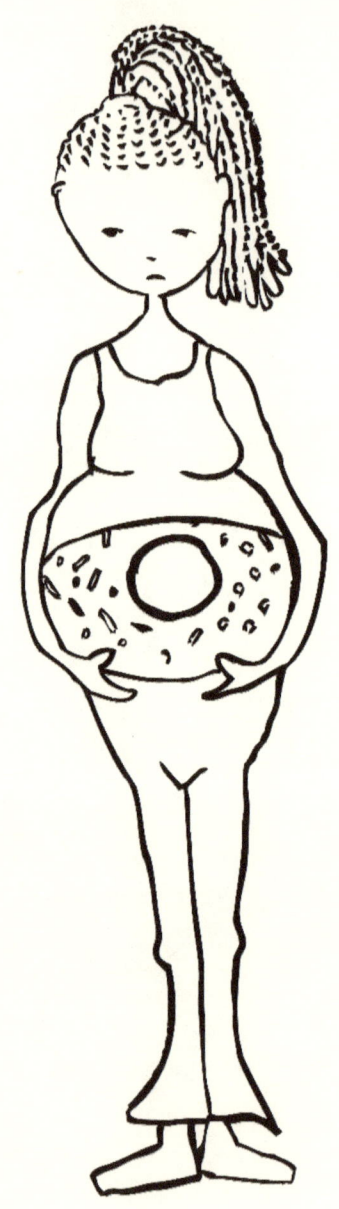

4

Julie Donut

Not many things in life compare to that wonderful feeling of eating. Let's face it. Eating is divine. Responding to the stomach-growling, mouth-watering anticipation of good food is one of life's greatest joys.

So why the angst?

Meet Julie.

Julie D.

7 a.m. The day starts off well after a little Oreo binge last night. The diet starts today. Just a piece of toast for breakfast and some coffee on the run.

10 a.m. Starving, standing in line at the coffee shop, a fresh donut beckons. NO. Must Resist. Have one of those bran muffins instead. The fiber will balance out the calories.

12 noon Appetite still sated after the muffin[4], Julie orders just a small salad for lunch. Yup. It's a Good Day.

4 p.m. Four hours later, famine strikes with hurricane force. MUST NOT EAT UNTIL DINNER. Okay. I'll have a coffee. 1 grande caramel soy macchiato, please. No whip.

6 p.m. Work day done. Back home in her kitchen, Julie faces a refrigerator full of vegetables from Saturday's farmers' market. First I'll have a drink, she says. Just 120 calories in 3 ounces of wine. Then a nice salad. Wait, I had that for lunch. What should I do with all these veggies? I'm hungry. Wonder what's in the freezer. Ice cream. No, no. What's this in here? A calorie-controlled Ready Meal? Oh barf.

---

[4] Your personal Julie Donut might substitute "a bag of chips" or "French fries" but you get the gist.

No, it's the right thing to do. Okay. Julie nukes the little frozen tray and pours another glass of wine. She carefully sets the table in front of the TV. Microwave beeps. She peels off the hot top and barely sits down. That label really should say, "Heat for three minutes, eat in 30 seconds." Dinner is done.

9 p.m. Three hours since that pathetic dinner. I've been SOooo good, Julie thinks, as her stomach rumbles. I'll microwave some popcorn. That's a low-cal snack. Beep. Munch munch stuff stuff. Bag empty by 9:30.

10:15 p.m. I'm kinda hungry. I won't be able to sleep. How about a tiny bowl of ice cream? One scoop. Okay, just a little more. And this? Licking the spoon doesn't really count. Yum – man, this is delicious. I'll have just a little more. *I deserve it, dammit. No one can tell me not to eat.* Now the carton's practically empty. I'd better eat the rest now – just to get rid of it. Remove all temptation so this *will never happen again.* Oh god, what am I doing?

11 p.m. No more ice cream. Julie brushes her teeth and falls into bed bloated, stuffed, ashamed, vowing once again to start her diet tomorrow.

Just a piece of toast for breakfast…
And so it continues.

Familiar?

Now imagine a different scenario. Same Julie, different last name.

Julie O.J.

7 a.m. Julie wakes up hungry. When she goes to the refrigerator, the first thing she sees is a chilled pitcher of orange juice. She pours a big glass, and drinks it as the coffee brews. The canister of oats beckons, and she makes herself a big bowl of oatmeal with fresh fruit and nuts, swimming in the sweet vanilla almond milk she picked up in the organic aisle. She fills her water bottle and heads out the door. At her desk, time flies until lunchtime.

12 noon Mmmmm, I'm so hungry…What shall I eat today? Julie O. goes to the local deli and gets a veggie wrap and a fresh smoothie. Eating feels SOooo good. She's stuffed.

4 p.m. A big cup of hot tea, then J.O. heads home.

6 p.m. Once home, Julie eats a juicy peach from the fruit bowl and thinks about what to have for dinner. Hmmm. What's in the freezer? Mmmm, those garlicky Tuscan Beans[5] she made last weekend. There are cut up veggies in the fridge, just waiting to be roasted. That sounds good. She pours a glass of wine, salts and seasons the veggies and pops them into the hot oven while she watches her favorite show. Her stomach growls as she smells the roasting vegetables.

---

[5] Recipe at end of book

6:30 p.m. Twenty minutes later, she nukes the beans, and fills the big plate with the roasted vegetables. It tastes SOooo good. Julie can't imagine anything more delightful than eating this delicious dinner. She eats as much as she wants. She even takes seconds.

9 p.m. Still satisfied, but wanting a little snack before she brushes her teeth, Julie enjoys a big handful of walnuts.

11 p.m. This was a good day, she thinks to herself before falling easily to sleep.

What is the difference here?

Julie Donut had 3,000 calories, felt guilty while she ate it and feels awful at the end of the day.
Julie Orange Juice had 1800 calories, ate all she wanted, whenever she wanted it, and felt great at the end of the day.
The Julies are both beautiful, perfect, intelligent women. Julie Donut spent the day fighting her hunger – and lost. Julie Orange Juice honored her appetite – and won.

Which one would you rather be?

5

Don't Torture Yourself

It was Thanksgiving. I had been married for less than a year and we were having dinner at my house. We invited friends (we'll call them the Ps) who graciously informed us ahead of time that they were following the Pritikin Diet.

This meant no fat.
No gravy.
No butter.
No problem, I thought.

I will roast the veggies without oil, and pass olive oil around for those who want it. Ditto for the potatoes and the gravy. And the peas with their cream sauce. Simple enough.

Also invited were our cousins (we'll call them the NPs) - epicureans who adored a feast. We told them about the P's requirements and they were fine with it. Fat optional. Check.

Drinks. Only water for the Ps. Champagne for the rest of us.

Dinnertime. Table set. Everything beautiful. Big steaming bowls on the glittering holiday table, full of:

Plain mashed potatoes. Boiled peas. Whole grain rolls. Whole roasted sweet potatoes.

Big vats of gravy and pats of butter sat shyly on a sideboard, there for the taking.

Everyone seemed happy, I thought.

Then dessert. I had made fruit cups for the Ps. Big juicy chunks of fruit – a bit hard to find in November. For the NPs and us, I had made a simple pecan pie with stealth whipped cream.

And guess what happened. Miss P accepted her pretty fruit cup. She set it before her, picked up a fork and stirred it around a little. She looked so sad. Then she took one look at the pecan pie - and a big smile crowded the frown off her starved face. She caved, quickly scarfing several pieces, whipped cream, guilt and all.

There's a moral here. Never torture yourself. And even more never: don't torture your hosts. This rule will come in very handy when you are eating at friends' houses. When they proudly pass the gooey rich brownies, *have one*. Lick it. Chew it. Love it. Honor it. By doing this, you will be satiated with one perfect serving, and will not feel guilty for it.[6]

The Olde You might think, "I blew it. I might as well give up for today anyway. I can start again tomorrow." But not the New You. The Newer, Smarter You knows that tomorrow never comes. Today is the day. Now is what matters. That brownie was absolutely delicious and there is absolutely no need to turn that beautiful thing into a binge. That would be silly.

A group of wonderful women I know have a name for this phenomenon. They call it *The All or Nothing Lizard*. It's that feeling that "I already messed up. Might as well eat the whole (cake/box/package/carton.)" But knowing about the Lizard makes it disappear. Diffuses its powers. Just kindly tell it to go outside and bother some other lizard, because you are *not interested*.

---

[6] (Of course, this does not apply if there are ingredients in said treat that will make you sick or compromise your compassion for animals and the earth.)

The more you truly love and honor your appetite,

the more you realize that the Good Stuff feels better.

And you can eat more of it, without guilt.

A Little Test for You

My Typical Weekday

I wake up

☐ singing	L
☐ and go running	S
☐ only long enough to hit the snooze button	A
☐ none of your business	C

The first thing I drink after getting out of bed is

☐ water	L
☐ something caffeinated	A
☐ juice	S
☐ none of your business	C

Next I have

☐ a nutritious breakfast, including whole grains	L
☐ a donut, pastry, something nice and sugary	A
☐ nothing	S
☐ none of your business	C

Two hours later, I

☐ need caffeine or sugar   A

☐ am hungry but I'll tough it out   S

☐ eat a small snack   L

☐ none of your business   C

Lunchtime. I

☐ eat a healthful, filling lunch   L

☐ nuke a prepackaged frozen diet lunch   S

☐ eat fast food   A

☐ none of your business   C

It's 4 p.m. I am

☐ eating sugar/sucking down caffeine   A

☐ eating a nutritious snack   L

☐ starving until dinnertime   S

☐ none of your business   C

Dinnertime. Finally. I

☐ scarf down some fast food or pizza   A

☐ eat a low calorie dinner   S

☐ eat everything in the refrigerator   A

☐ eat a perfectly nutritious balanced dinner   L

☐ don't do anything (a.k.a. none of your business)   C

In the hours before bed, I usually

- [ ] eat a light snack   L
- [ ] don't eat – only tea for me   S
- [ ] eat (or drink) about half my daily calories A
- [ ] eat (or drink) even more than that   A
- [ ] none of your business   C

INTERPRETING YOUR RESULTS:

Mostly Ls: You are Perfect. A Goddess of Good Eating. Bravo. Give this book away immediately. (Unless, of course, you're lying.)

Mostly Ss: You are *A Dieter*. You don't love your body if you're starving it. Relax! Eat!

Mostly As: How's this working for you? Oh? That's why you're reading this book?

All Cs: Touche. Give this book to someone else.

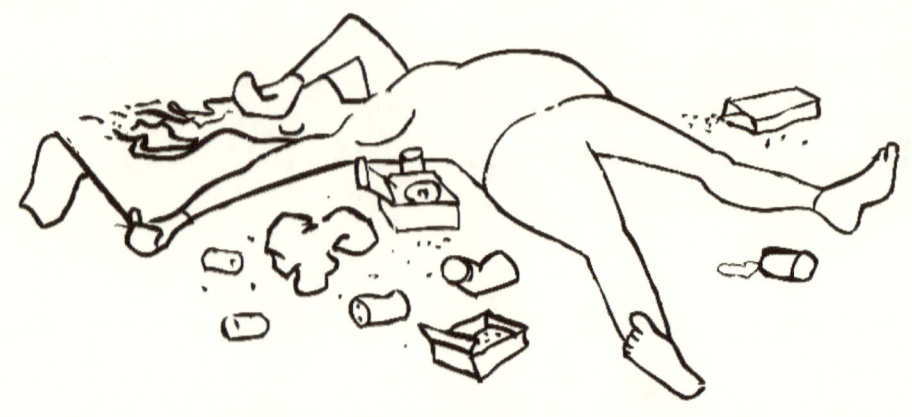

MOSTLY Ls, Ss or As?

The way I see it, you have three choices:

GIVE UP (AND GET FATTER)

FIGHT (AND GET MADDER)

RELAX (AND SUCCEED)

You already know how to do the first two.
Before you've finished reading this,
you'll know how to do the last one.

6

Desire

You are probably reading this book because you have been challenged by your desires. Desire is a complicated thing. You might desire health. You might desire wealth, happiness, fitness. (Now you also might desire a piece of pecan pie. Sorry.)
Are these desires mutually exclusive? Yeah, probably. Pie will not make you rich, happy, fit or healthy. But that doesn't mean you don't still crave it.

Centered in your brain's most ancient, wonderfully fabulous limbic system,[7] desire evolved to keep you alive, by compelling you to seek

---

[7] See chapter 9

elements necessary to survival: water (thirst), food (hunger), sex (procreation), safety (fight or flight.)

This all worked fine when we were cave people. Drink, eat, procreate, fight, run. That about covered it. But desire became more complicated as we evolved. While original desires for survival were interchangeable with needs, as humans conquered those needs, strange yearnings emerged.

We developed desire for sheer entertainment. Eating and drinking became social. Sex became recreational more than procreational. *It is rumored that some humans even learned to run for fun and not fear.* All exaggerated needs, not necessary for survival now, but just as powerful.

So here we are a zillion years later, full of desires that feel very real, but…are they?

When Buddha said that desire is the cause of all suffering, I suspect he was speaking of the modern human.

Modern, unnecessary desire = Bad.

Caveman desire = Good.

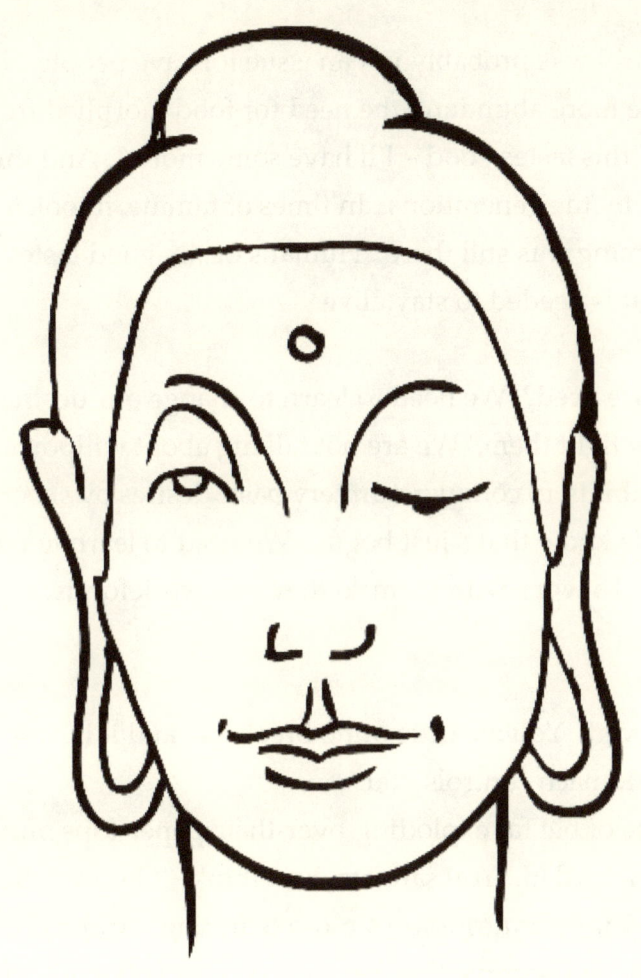

Weight control was probably not an issue for cave people. Then as food became more abundant, the need for food morphed from survival to "this tastes good – I'll have some more." And this new desire grew by the generations. In times of famine, it took a back seat, but the yearning was still there. Humans desire good tastes – way beyond what is needed to stay alive.

So what *do* we need? We need to learn to change our desires. By this I don't mean fight them. We are not talking about willpower – that impossible ability to conquer our very basic desires by sheer mental strength. We know that's just bogus. We need to learn to reprogram our desires. To work with them so they will work for us.

Imagine this:
You are starved. You ate little or no breakfast, and it is now hours later. Your stomach controls you.
Enter: a plate of big fat exploding-over-their-paper-tops muffins, and a huge spinach salad. You salivate. You think, "I know I should eat the salad." But the muffins are s-o-o-o tempting. And so easy to eat. And after all, you deserve this, because you haven't eaten much all day. "I'll have the salad next time," you tell yourself, as you reach for a muffin.

Now imagine this:
You are hungry. You feel the familiar growl in your empty stomach that reminds you who's really in charge. Your stomach controls you.

Enter: two plates. One is a huge spinach salad. The other is piled high with – yup – explodingly delicious-looking muffins.
You AUTOMATICALLY reach for the salad not because you are super-strong, not because of "willpower," but because you TRULY want the salad, and not the muffin. The muffins look kinda good, but *the salad is what triggers your watering mouth.*

What? You're kidding, right?

Curtain closes. Shuffle shuffle. Curtain rises.

Take I: You sit bloated, stuffed full of muffins. You didn't stop at one, even. You scarfed two in record time and now you feel…good? No. You feel stuffed. Guilty. "Why did I do that?" you ask yourself. And your self answers: "because your brain told you the muffins would taste better than the salad, and that made your mouth water, and that made your hand reach out and grab the muffin. Duh."

Curtain closes. Shuffle shuffle. Curtain rises.

Take II: Your stomach is full. You feel SO good. That spinach salad was absolutely delicious, from first bite to last. You are ready for your close up. Maybe you'll have a muffin later.

You're probably thinking, there's NO way. This might work for someone else, but not me. I'm a carbs addict. I hate spinach. No WAY would I choose the salad over the muffin. This book sucks.

Okay. Quit reading then.

Because you aren't going to believe what I have to tell you now.

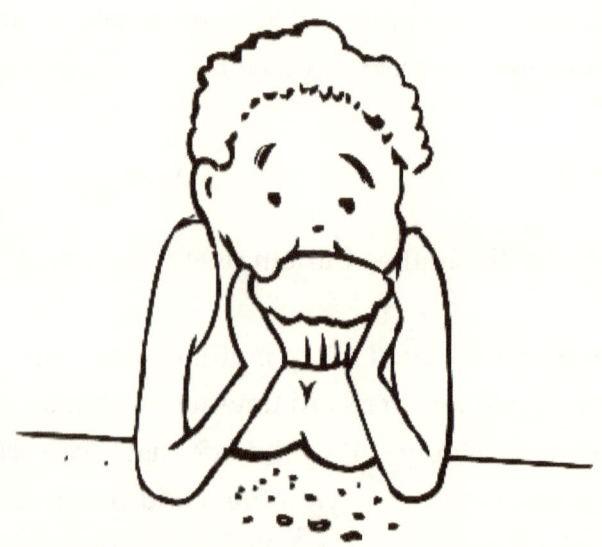

WITH VERY LITTLE WORK,
EVEN MUFFIN PEOPLE CAN BE REFORMED.

I don't mean "develop willpower" or learn some super strength to deflect muffins. I mean you will be totally, 100 percent CHANGED, so that the good foods become *what you truly desire*, and the extra treats become just that. Treats.

LimbaSlim is a permanent solution. You will become a person who truly loves good foods. And a person who eats absolutely all she wants, without guilt, calorie counting, or any of that usual b.s. that we know doesn't work.

I am not kidding.

Read on.

7

Cheating

Few things feel better than a perfectly full tummy. We eat not only when we're hungry for nutrition, but for security - for that comforting blanket of wellbeing that comes from satiation. Mommies everywhere encourage their babies to eat, eat, eat. They smile when baby eats. They get frustrated when she won't. From our very first nursings, filling our stomachs is accompanied by the deepest, most profound love of our lives.

But what about skinny people?
Skinny people drank from the same sweet, tempting breast – but they eat when they are hungry for nutrition, not for comfort. And they stop eating when their stomachs are full. Surely they need comfort

too. Is it possible that they get it elsewhere, and not from food? Like from happy memories? Like from dear friends and close family? Like from keeping active and using food only as body fuel and social play?

Yup. That's what they do. And the irony is that by eating this way – by listening to and respecting their stomachs - naturally slim people easily fit "forbidden" treats into their plan without going overboard. When we see a skinny person scarfing down a big dessert, we think, "Hey, that's just not fair. If I ate that..." But skinny people aren't ashamed of their eating, so they can do it in public – actually **eating whatever they feel like eating**! Imagine that.

No, really. IMAGINE that. Because even if it sounds corny: *if we imagine it, we can be it.* If advertising can implant negative self-esteem, we can just as easily implant good self-esteem. They're *our* brains. Let's take them back.

There will be no such thing as cheating any more. When you have finished here - and you have changed your desires - you will be eating healthfully by CHOICE. If you decide to treat yourself with something decidedly "not healthful," you will enjoy it thoroughly and easily stop with one serving. Or maybe less. No guilt.

It is a whole new mindset. Say you are going out for drinks and dinner. Before LimbaSlim, you would probably have worried about "going off my diet." Or (a little better) maybe you would be saying, "Screw this. I deserve to treat myself. No calorie counting tonight!"

Now you will not have to give either of these notions a second thought. You will go out. You will order exactly what you want, and eat/drink as much as you want of it. But WHAT YOU WANT will be different.

Once I was telling the Muffin v. Spinach story to a small audience. When I came to the part about, "of course you WANT the muffin" a woman called out, "No, not me. I would way rather have the salad." I could hear from her voice that she was sincere (not a sarcastic heckler) I looked toward the voice, and wasn't surprised to see that she was a slim gray-haired woman. Happy, trim, fit looking. I asked her, "Have you always been thin?" and she said, "Yes. I just don't like crappy food."
This woman was born with the LimbaSlim mentality. We might not be so lucky. But we can change it.

(A Little Aside About Alcohol)
Sometimes a girl's just gotta party. I know this isn't what I'm supposed to say here, but it's my book, and I believe in having fun.

[If you are a recovering alcoholic, I apologize for this and send you all my admiration, love and strength.]

If you go out for drinks, it's hard to drink club soda. So, what should you order?

I personally think martinis are the answer, and here's why:

Martinis have the most bang for the calorie buck and they don't have nasty sulfites or additives. Granted, they have no nutritional value, but if you have been eating only good stuff all week, you've had plenty of vitamins already. So go ahead, have a martini. [8] You will very likely notice that you won't even want more than one. I know this sounds improbable to some of you, but once your body is used to the good stuff you're putting in it, it might not handle the bad stuff quite the same way. So one martini. Two if you're nuts. And not every day.

---

[8] or a shot of tequila, or vodka on the rocks, or a shot of whisky like in Deadwood. But just one. Please consult your doctor, regardless.

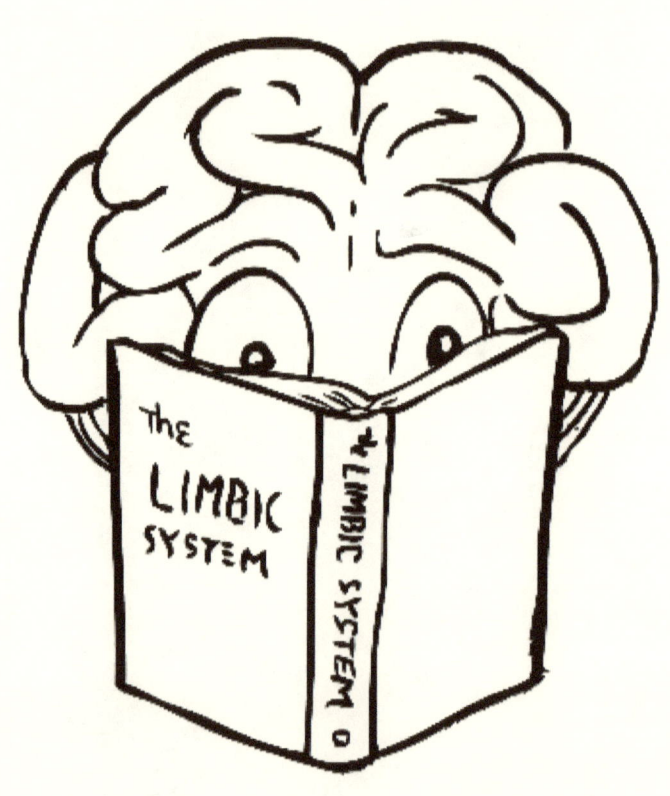

8

Your Groovy Brain

The human brain has approximately 100 billion neurons. Neurons - the cells in the central nervous system - collect information from the eyes, skin, nose, tongue, and ears and send it to the brain. Information flows from one neuron to another over pathways called synapses. When the same message is continually fired down a synapse, the route it takes becomes "grooved" into the brain. It's kind of like a trail. The more it gets walked on, the more it becomes a permanent path. We call it learning.

For example, a baby takes her first steps. Nerves fire between sensors in her feet, her inner ear, her muscles. At first, she is clumsy; the brain synapses are new. Eventually, as she repeats the motions of walking, the synapses get used to the path, and eventually walking becomes an unconscious skill.

Synapses are involved in our lives as adults, too. We are affected every day by our experiences. When an experience is repeated enough, it becomes grooved into our brains' synaptic paths. Of course millions of pathways are formed when we are infants, but science now knows that the brain continues to create new synapses all our lives.

Which is all fine when it comes to habits we want and need. The problem comes when it applies to habits we wish to change.

A smoker is a good example. The first time he lights up, there are no synapses established for this new sensation, so the newly-affected sensory neurons create a new and awkward path. As he continues smoking, pleasure centers light up in the brain's limbic system, rewarding this new synaptic journey. As it is repeated again and again, the paths are strengthened, until smoking tobacco becomes an unconscious habit, perhaps no longer so pleasurable, but ingrained just the same.

Eating is like this. Imagine a newborn human being's first meal: Breast milk is sweet. It comes with close touching and a feeling of warmth and safety that become forever linked in the brain. The path is established with great reward and fanfare. It's no wonder that eating feels so good. But for some of us, the brain seems to have made the deduction that if a full stomach is good, a fuller one is even better. And this is the bit we can change.

There are very few ways a mind path can be altered. One is by physical brain damage, which is not recommended. And the other is through mental accessing of the subconscious mind by working with the programmable brainwave states and *showing the brain a new path.* That new path must be tread again and again until it becomes the pathway of choice deep within your groovy brain.

If repeated exposure to advertising and supermodels can screw up our eating so thoroughly, doesn't it make sense that we can screw it back down again by repeating more helpful messages?

We need help - to reprogram the brain, to create new mind paths that tell the body it is beautiful, secure, and safe. We need to get access to our own limbic systems. That help comes to you via your nose.

Our sense of smell, or olfaction, is the one sense in the human body that is directly connected to the brain. The olfactory bulb provides a straight channel between the outside world and the brain's limbic system - the ancient center of memory, emotion, desire and addiction. This phenomenon - the connection between the sense of smell and the ancient limbic system – is the key to the power of LimbaSlim.

9

The Limbic System

This most ancient part of your brain is responsible for pleasure, addiction, memory, pride, orgasm, eating.

By Jove, I think we're onto something.

LimbaSlim will work for you whether or not you know which part of your brain is lighting up when you use it. Nevertheless, I feel compelled to share with you some basic information about your very cool limbic system.

It may well be boring, but as a funny friend of mine assured me, "You can only make neuroscience so peppy."

Our bodies are comprised of a variety of different systems:

- The endocrine system contains glands and controls hormones and whatnot.
- The excretory system takes care of all the stuff that needs to come out of us.
- The immune system fights invading diseases.
- The integumentary system is a fancy word for skin.
- The nervous system has the nerves.
- The reproductive system makes babies.
- The respiratory system handles our oxygen.
- The skeletal and muscular systems hold it all together.

But the greatest of these – for our purposes here – is the limbic system.

The limbic system is a part of the nervous system (that means the brain and spinal cord) that sits in the deepest part of the brain. The limbic system is sometimes called the reptilian brain, because it is very very old, like lizards.

One might assume that the limbic system is the reason we evolved at all. It is the system that gives us pleasure (not just us, but all animals) so that we know to keep on eating and reproducing. Sometimes referred to as the "emotional brain," the limbic system is responsible for processing and storing memory, fear, sex drive and emotion. It is the processing center for addictions, *including overeating*, and is the part of the brain that reacts to a recently-discovered protein called leptin, which is released by fat cells when we overeat.

Key Parts of the Limbic System

The most prominent parts of the limbic system are the amygdala, hypothalamus, and hippocampus.

Amygdala

The amygdalas are two almond-shaped masses of neurons that appear to control the sex drive, fear and aggression.

Hypothalamus

The hypothalamus is the biggie. It is responsible for regulating hunger, thirst, response to pain, anger and aggression, pulse, blood pressure, breathing, and sexual arousal.

Hippocampus

The hippocampus consists of two "horns" that curve back from the amygdala. It is responsible for processing memory and converting short term memories to long term.

The limbic system is an old term, and current science has blurred the lines between "inside" and "outside" it. Sometimes included are the *cingulated gyrus, the septum, the ventral tegmental area, the prefrontal cortex and the basal ganglia.* I include these here not only because I don't want to leave anyone out, but because I actually hope some neuroscientists will read this book and call me up, to praise my brilliant, lay-friendly descriptions.

If you had to choose your favorite brain part, I would definitely suggest choosing the limbic system. It was there for us when we were lizards – rewarding behavior that kept us alive. Our sense of smell, directly connected to the limbic system via the olfactory bulb, was probably the most important sense at one time. We smelled rotten food. We smelled enemy B.O. We smelled pheromones that led us to our true lizard loves.

Over the millennia, however, we have gotten blasé about smell. Ask anyone which sense they'd rather give up: sight, hearing, or smell, and they will usually choose smell. I know this because I asked at least five people. But the truth is, if you REALLY lost your sense of smell, you would be very sad.

Smell is the only one of our senses that is directly connected to our brains.

So thank you, limbic system.
Thank you, olfactory bulb.
Thank you, LimbaSniffer.

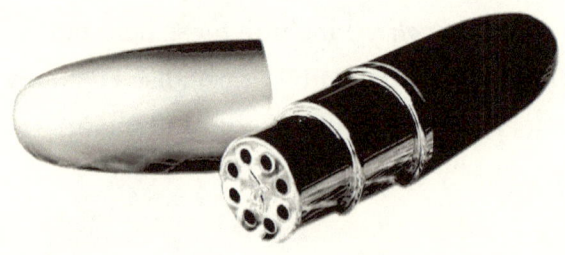

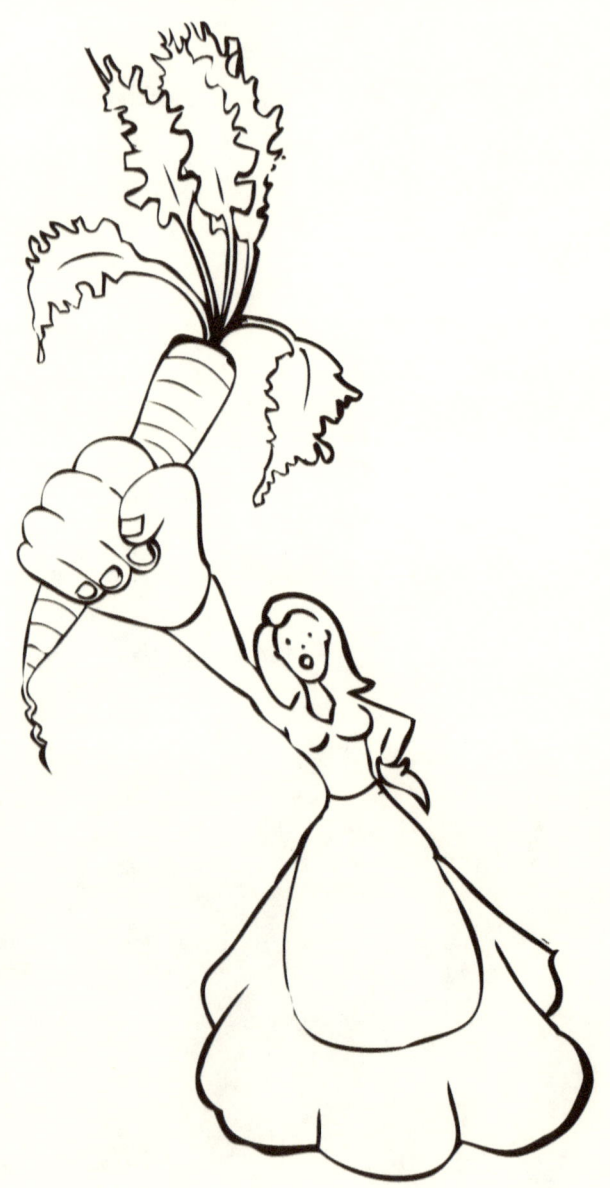

10

CLOSE TO THE EARTH

THE GIST

Eating Close to the Earth is a simple guideline that will help your body, your soul, and the planet. Once you are used to it, you will never want to eat another way. Because probably for the first time since infancy, *you will be eating as much and as often as you want.*

The only requirement is that the foods you eat are grown from the earth and are as unprocessed as possible.

The premise is that when you feed your body only natural foods, it will eat until satisfied to establish its ideal weight and stay there.

It's very simple. Feed your body as it's been asking to be fed all along. You will feel better than you have ever felt, with more energy and a newfound self pride as your weight drops steadily. Eventually, most people find their weight stabilizes, which is a sign that they have reached their personal goal – the weight that is perfect for their own body.

THE LIST

Just in case you're thinking this means you can only eat carrot sticks forever, here's a little list of some of what you'll be eating. You will eat *all you want* from the list on these pages.

(A Sample Daily Menu follows the list.)

Acorn squash

Almond butter

Apples

Apricots

Artichoke

Asparagus

Avocados

Bamboo shoots

Barley

Beans, all kinds: dry or canned

Beet greens

Beets

Bell pepper

Black beans

Blackberries

Black-eyed peas

Blueberries

Bok choy

Brazil nuts

Broad beans

Broccoli

Brown rice

Brussels sprouts

Bulgur (cracked wheat)

Butter beans

Cabbage

Calico beans

Cannellini beans

Cantaloupe

Carrots

Casaba melon

Cashews

Cauliflower

Celery

Cereal: whole grain*

Cherries

Chickpeas

Chicory

Chili pepper

Chinese cabbage

Chives

Collard greens

Crackers: like Rye Krisp or Wasa Krisp*

Cranberries

Crenshaw

Cress

Currants

Dandelion greens

Edamame

Eggplant

Endive

Escarole

Fava beans

Fennel

Filberts

Flax

Garbanzo beans

Garlic

Ginger

Grains

Grapes

Great northern beans

Green beans

Greens

Guacamole

Hazelnut butter

Hazelnuts

Honeydew

Hummus

Jicama

Kale

Kidney beans

Kiwi fruit

Kohlrabi

Kumquats

Leek

Lentils

Lettuce

Lima beans

Melons

Millet

Mustard greens

Napa cabbage

Navy beans

Nectarines

Nut butters

Nuts

Oatmeal

Oats

Okra

Onions

Parsley

Parsnips

Peaches

Peanut butter

Peanuts

Pears

Peas

Peppers: red, green, yellow and hot

Persimmons

Pinto beans

Pistachios

Plums

Pomegranates

Potatoes

Prunes

Pumpkin

Pumpkin seeds

Quinoa

Radicchio

Radish

Raisins

Raspberries

Refried beans (vegetarian)

Rutabaga

Rye

Rye Krisp crackers*

Salsa

Salsify

Sesame seeds

Shallot

Soybeans

Spinach

Split peas

Squash

Steel cut oats

Strawberries

Summer squash

Sunflower seeds

Sweet peppers

Sweet potato

Tomatoes

Tortillas – whole grain and corn*

Turnips

Walnut butter

Walnuts

Wasa Krisp*

Water chestnut

Wheat berries

White Beans

Wild rice
Winter squash
Yams
Zucchini

*EXTRAS:
Condiments (mustard, ketchup, Asian condiments, chutneys, etc.)
Curry
Hot sauce
Soy sauce
Tofu
Vinaigrette
Olive oil and other nutritious oils
Whole grain cold cereals
Soy/nut/rice milks
Coffee, tea
Dark chocolate (70% cacao)

(*Add in **Extras** as you wish. If you think any of them will cause you to overeat, don't use them. Salt is okay unless your doctor says otherwise. Ditto for coffee and tea. Alcohol: see Chapter 7.)

When you wake each morning, you will look forward to the delicious day ahead of you - no more dieting or obsessing about food and calories. At first it will be challenging, but that's where your LimbaSniffer comes in.

NOTE: Even if you don't have the LimbaSlim system, you can certainly follow this plan. Some people need the help LimbaSlim offers, but some won't. And it's a plan your whole family can adopt – even the skinny ones.

"DIETING"

There is no measuring or counting with this plan.
Most women find they lose a pound a week consistently,
sometimes much more, especially in the beginning.
IF you really want to lose weight faster, you can of course use
this same list, but also count calories.
Don't go below 1500 calories a day. Please.
Because that is torture, which we've already covered.

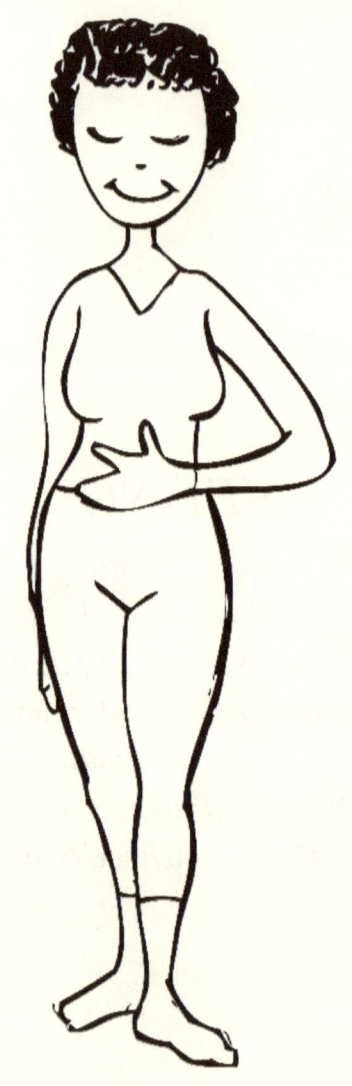

A SAMPLE DAILY MENU

Breakfast:

A big bowl of hot or cold **whole grain cereal**, with **blueberries, sliced banana** and almond milk.
Coffee or tea
Big glass of water or juice

Lunch:

Huge green salad with everything and vinaigrette
Veggie bean soup **(recipe)**
Big **nectarine**
Big glass of water

Dinner:

Pile up:

2 corn **tortillas**

Guacamole (recipe)

Refried beans

Lettuce or other greens

Salsa (recipe or bought)

Big glass of water

Snacks (anytime):

Bowl of frozen **blueberries**

Fresh **fruit smoothie** (recipe)

Baby spinach salad

Crispy cold **red peppers** dipped in **hummus (recipe)**

Rye Krisp with **peanut butter**

Apple slices with **peanut butter**

Handful of **raw almonds or walnuts**

Sunflower seeds in the shell

Coffee/tea

NOTE: If you ate everything on the Sample Daily Menu, you would
have consumed 1,932 calories and 53 grams of protein. You probably

won't ever eat this much. But you can if you want to. Here are some other nutrient values from the menu above[9]:

NUTRIENTS:	RDA[10]	SAMPLE MEAL
Calories:	2300	1932
Calcium:	100-150 mg	145
Iron:	100-150 mcg	159
Protein:	50 grams	53
*Vitamin A:	800 ue	1590
Vitamin B-6:	100-200 mg	245
*Vitamin C:	100 mg	876
*Vitamin E:	100 mg	100
Zinc:	100-200 mg	165
Potassium:	100 mg	700
Fiber:	25-35 grams	47

*ANTIOXIDANTS

Protein percentages in some plant foods

---

[9] from Sparkpeople.com – what a phenomenal website

[10] RDAs are based on a 160-pound woman over 35 who is moderately active

Soybean sprouts	54
Spinach	49
Broccoli	45
Kale	45
Mung bean sprouts	43
Cauliflower	40
Bamboo shoots	39
Mushrooms	38
Chinese cabbage	34
Lettuce	34
Wheat germ	31
Zucchini	28
Navy beans	26
Cabbage	22
Pumpkin seeds	21
Whole wheat	17
Lemons	16
Oats	15
Walnuts	13
Honeydew melon	10
Brown rice	8
Strawberries/oranges/cherries/apricots/watermelon/grapes	8
Pecans	5

It's colorful, eating this way.
And you will absolutely love it.

As Goddess is my witness,
you will never be hungry again[11]!

---

[11] Sorry, Scarlet

11

Today is the First Day of the Rest of Your Life

Yes, I really named this chapter that.

Having read this far, I figure that you are convinced, and finally free of the shackles of Unrealistic Blockheaded Anti-woman Body Expectations. (U-BABE.)

You are free of the tyranny of dieting. Forever.

But, uh, now what?

The first thing to do is to get rid of all the stuff in your kitchen that doesn't fit the criterion in Chapter 10. Here are some ideas on how to best and most appropriately rid your refrigerator and cabinets of Junk, in reverse order of preference.

1. Eat it all tonight.
2. Give it to a friend who hasn't read this book.
3. Compost it.
4. Send it to the television network you feel is the most egregious in U-BABE promotion.

SHOPPING

Next, go shopping. If you're cooking for yourself only, you really won't need a trip to Costco for ten pounds of red peppers. Take your reusable bags, and head for the small local health food stores and co-ops. Wander the farmers' markets. By shopping locally, you support local farms, reduce your carbon footprint, lessen your personal chemical load, and sometimes even see your food's source.

COOKING

Now go make some stuff. There are recipes in the back of the book, and sources for even more online and in some wonderful blogs and cookbooks. Google earth-friendly cooking, eating local, slow food movement.

EATING

Eat all you want, but only foods that are Close to the Earth. If you're dining out, ask yourself, "Did someone grow this?" (Test tubes don't count.)

During the first week, you may feel as if you are overeating. But remember, *there is no such thing as cheating anymore.* Eat ALL you want. Don't stifle yourself. It will all even out as you get more used to this delicious whole foods way of eating. THERE IS NO GUILT ALLOWED. EVER. That said, don't go crazy just to prove me wrong. That would just be dumb.

You will be honoring your appetite, and believe me, it will feel great. When your stomach growls for food, give it FOOD. All you want. Real food.

Listen to your LimbaSlim meditation every day, and carry your LimbaSniffer with you.

Now run along. You have shopping, cooking and eating to do.

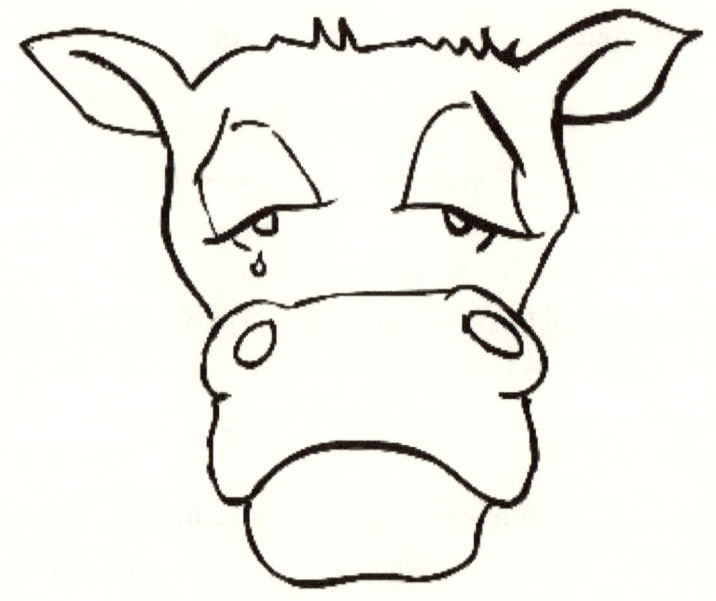

12

Please Don't
Eat the Poodles

Have you heard the urban myth about the woman whose dog is accidentally cooked and served to her in a foreign restaurant? It totally put me off poodle.

Horrified? Continue if you dare. If you are already sensitive to animal issues, please skip this chapter.

What I can't understand is why anyone would want to eat any animal - be it poodle, horse, cow, pig, chicken. They're all sentient beings.

Each species has been someone's friend, some child's pet. So in this chapter, I beg you: please don't eat the poodles.

At this point, you are probably thinking one of the following:

"YAY for the animals. But don't make me read this."
"Wait. I need my protein."
"F*** you. I just want to lose weight. Spare me the sermon, you animal rights activist you."

These reactions are okay. Well, except for the last two. Please bear with me.[12] And don't read the following if you don't eat meat. You know this story already, and it is sad.

I just want to ask you:

When you drive by those sweet cows in pastures across America, do you think, "What's the fuss about? They live lovely – dare I say bucolic – lives. I wouldn't mind standing in a grassy field all day with my friends, nothing to do but eat. Then boom, dead, hamburger. It ain't a bad gig."

---

[12] Mmmmmmmm, bear…

Do you really think this is what it is like?
Let's follow one cow. We'll call her Ferdie.

[The following story is based on information from the cattle industry.]

Ferdie is born in a spring green pasture in the middle of Oklahoma. Her mother, Sue, licks her clean as she takes her first stand on wobbly calf legs. Ferdie finds Mama's udder and has a nice warm meal before settling down to nap in the lush grass. The rest of the herd comes around to welcome Ferdie. They stand there dopey-looking, watching with big brown eyes and chewing their cuds as the newest family member sleeps.

Ferdie's life is simple. After about a week, she learns to eat grass. She plays and romps with the other calves - her friends. As the summer wanes, the farmer brings them big piles of hay. Winter offers new fun, playing in the snow, but when it melts, and spring comes, things begin to change. First Ferdie gets a metal tag put in her ear. The tagging hurts a little, but castration for her male friends is way worse.

Castration is the removal of the testicles of bull calves "to reduce meat toughness, aggressive behavior, sexual interest and dark cutting." (from cattlenetwork.com/Cattle_Preconditioning.) There are several ways this is done. Sometimes it is done at birth. But Ferdie's farmer thought it was nicer to castrate her friends another way, after they were a little bit older. If Ferdie could read, she would know that it was their misfortune to be born American cattle. In most countries, castration is always preceded by an injection that numbs the area.

Not here. Ferdie's farmer and his friends come in one morning, ready to start. One by one, the men grab the male calves and quickly snap a thick rubber band tight around their scrota. A few days later, the pain starts - also the smell, as the boys' testicles rot and finally fall off.

When Ferdie is about six months old, she and her friends are herded onto a big truck. They cry out for their mothers. The truck is crowded, dark, smelly and very hot. The animals are afraid. There is no water. One of Ferdie's friends lies down and doesn't want to get up.

When the truck finally stops, the calves are let out. There are men waiting for them. These men don't have hay. They have electric cattle prods, which hurt.

Ferdie is really scared now. There is a lot of noise. This isn't normal. This isn't right. Why won't some of her friends get up? Where is her mother?

There are hundreds of calves in this new place, called a feedlot. There is no more grass now, no room to run or play. The feedlot is dirty and muddy, with a lot of food in big containers. Ferdie and her friends don't eat or drink anything for the first few days. A few of them fall down in the mud. When they don't get up, the men drag them away. But finally the survivors learn to eat and drink with the huge rubbing crowd of cows. There are flies everywhere - they seem to like the open wounds the cows get from bumping into one another and the feeding troughs.

Ferdie's weight doubles in the six months she lives in the feedlot. Then one day, some men come to the lot with their cattle prods again.

Ferdie and the other cows are herded out of the feedlot and into a wooden chute. One by one, a man points a gun at their heads. BANG. A calf falls down on his knees, but is quickly hung up with rope by his hind legs. Another man cuts his throat so the blood can drain out. Another man begins cutting off his skin.

Ferdie is watching this. The air is filled with cries of terror. Her friends are panicking - they poop all over - it is hell. Then it's Ferdie's turn. People really like hamburgers.

Back in the pasture at home, the mother cows welcome Ferdie's little brother into the herd as another lovely, bucolic life begins.

What about Free Range?

All I can suggest here is that you look into it thoroughly before chowing down. Have you visited a "free range" chicken farm? I did this once, and was overwhelmed by the horrendously crowded barn, the stench of ammonia. The chickens did have outdoor access: one tiny door, but they didn't go out. If you're thinking, "See? Chickens are dumb," I can only wonder if that means you feel you should eat them. Because if that's the criterion for edibility, I know some free range politicians you might find tasty.

**One large unadorned baked potato
has as much protein as 100 calories of meat.**

MORE PROTEIN FACTS

You need 20 to 50 grams of protein a day. There is no difference
nutritionally in animal and vegetable protein. The biggest animals
are vegetarians. A human being doubles its weight in its first 6
months of life, during which it is typically consuming a diet that is
0.8% to 0.9% protein (breast milk), and no meat. Breast milk in
vegetarian mothers has protein content equal to meat-eating mothers.

Protein in grams in 100 calories of beef: 9

Protein in grams in 100 calories of cheese: 6

Protein in grams in 100 calories of broccoli : 45

LEGAL DISCLAIMER

Ask your doctor before starting any new eating plan.

*We've all heard that doctors learn zip about nutrition in college.
If yours says you must eat meat, find another one. Stat.*

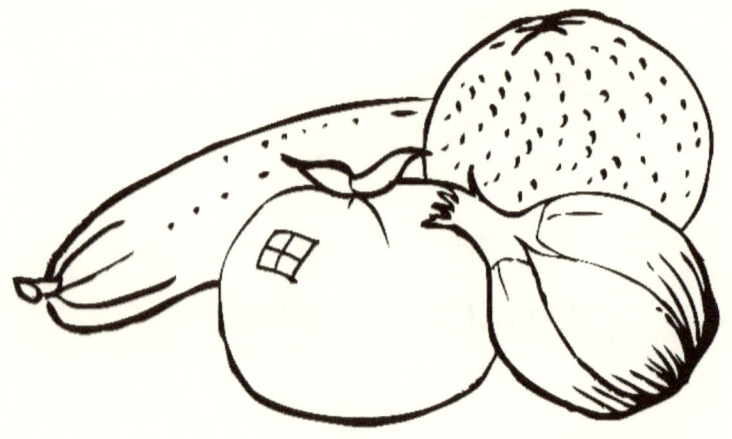

RECIPES
A Little Easy Cooking

CREAMY TUSCAN BEANS

(Start the night before)

2 c dry white beans (cannellini, Great Northern, or navy)

2-3 c hot water

2 T olive oil

3-4 sage leaves or 1 t. dry sage

2-3 cloves garlic, chopped

Salt

Pepper

Directions: Start the night before. Soak beans in cold water to cover for at least 8 hours (use lots of water so they don't ever get dry.) Rinse well and drain.

Preheat oven to 325 F. Place beans in casserole dish and add very hot tap water to cover by 1 inch. Add oil, sage, and garlic. Cover pan tightly with aluminum foil and poke 6 pencil-sized holes in it. Bake for 2-3 hours until tender and creamy. You will know when they're done when the liquid is truly creamy, not watery. Add salt at the end. (This is important: *if you salt beans before cooking, they won't cook!*)

GOOD OLD HUMMUS

2 cups cooked garbanzo beans or chickpeas (see cooking method on

page 115) or 1 can, drained and thoroughly rinsed.

2 cloves garlic

2 T. lemon juice

2T. olive oil

1 T. tahini

Salt to taste (1/4 t. or so)

A tiny bit of water if necessary to make it smooth.

Directions: Mash the heck out of all these ingredients - either use a ricer, a food processor, a blender, a potato masher or a fork. Make as smooth as possible. Store in fridge.

 Makes about 2 cups.

EGGPLANT DIP - AKA Baba Ghanoush

1 large or 2 medium eggplant(s)

2 garlic cloves, crushed

2 T. tahini (sesame paste)

1/4 cup scallions, finely chopped

Juice of one lemon

1/4 cup chopped parsley

salt

paprika (optional)

Directions: Preheat oven to 400 degrees. Prick eggplant all over with a fork. Place in oven for 45-50 minutes until very soft. Remove from oven, allow to cool. Scoop out soft flesh from eggplant, and mash with garlic, tahini, scallions, lemon juice and parsley. (Or use blender or food processor on pulse - you don't want this totally pureed, but a little chunky.) Refrigerate until ready to serve. Great with raw veggies.

Makes 2 cups.

SALSA FRESCA

Cut up five ripe tomatoes (in winter, plum tomatoes are best)

Toss with 1 T. lemon or lime juice

1/2 small onion, diced

a splash of hot sauce, a shake of cayenne or chopped hot chilies to

taste

1/2 t. salt (or less)

Optional: 1/2 bunch of chopped cilantro (some like this flavor, some

don't)

Mix by hand, not in food processor or it will get all bubbly.
Store in fridge up to 5 days. Serve with raw veggies for dipping, or
use in wholegrain tortilla with refried bean recipe below.
Makes about 2 cups.

DIRTY BEAN DIP

1 can vegetarian refried beans

2 cloves garlic, crushed

1 T. olive oil

1/2 t. salt

1 T. lime or lemon

1 t. chili powder or 1/2 t. cumin

Mix well. Store covered in fridge. Use as dip with raw vegetables, or as yummy filling for wholegrain burrito.
Makes about 2 cups.

BASIC GUACAMOLE

Smashed up ripe avocado - just peel and smash it in a bowl with a fork.

1 T. lemon or lime juice

(optional) 2 T. diced onion, 1 diced tomato

1/8 t. salt or less to taste

Cayenne pepper or hot sauce or chopped hot chilies to taste.

Great as a dip for fresh raw veggies.

Makes about 1 cup.

SOUPER DOUPER VEGETABLE SOUP

1 large onion, coarsely chopped

2 huge carrots or 1/2 bag baby carrots, chopped as desired

5 stalks celery, leaves and all, cut in small slices

2 cloves garlic, peeled and chopped or smashed

1 quart Vegetarian broth

1 15-oz. can diced tomatoes (or 3 chopped fresh tomatoes)

olive oil

salt

bunch kale leaves or other greens, chopped

hot sauce (Tabasco-like)

In largest deep stovetop pan or Dutch oven on medium heat, heat 1 T. olive oil and toss vegetables in, except for garlic up. When onion is translucent, add chopped garlic and stir. Immediately pour in 1 quart of veggie broth

Add diced tomatoes, 1 t. salt, and herbs to your heart's content (suggestions: sage or rosemary) Add hot sauce to taste. Bring to boil, then turn down and cook on low simmer for 30 minutes or more. You can also put this in the crock pot on high for 4 hours or low for 8 hours.

Add the chopped greens when reheating, or in the last 10 minutes of cooking. This soup gets better and better as the hours and days go by. You can add virtually any vegetable you like, except potatoes, which will turn the whole soup mushy after a while. Lima beans, garbanzos, anything you like that comes from the earth.

Makes about 8 cups.

SIMPLE SPEEDY BEAN SOUP

large onion

2 cloves garlic

1 green pepper

2 cups vegetable broth

1 can or 2 cups (cooked) kidney beans

1 can vegetarian or fat free refried beans

Salt, pepper, hot sauce

Olive oil

Chili power or cumin

Lemon or lime juice

In largest deep stovetop pan/ Dutch oven on medium heat, heat 1 T. olive oil and toss in 1 chopped onion. Add 1 T. chili powder or 1 t. cumin. When onion is translucent, add chopped garlic and stir - don't burn the garlic! Immediately pour in 2 cups veggie broth plus 1 T.

lemon or lime juice. Stir in 1 can refried beans, 1 can (or 2 cups precooked) kidney beans. Mix well, add 2 t. salt (or to taste) and cook until just heated through. This soup gets better and better as it sits in the fridge.

Makes about 7 cups.

MAKE IT INTO CHILI: Add 5 cloves of garlic, minced, 3 jalapeno peppers, minced and 1 15-oz. can crushed tomatoes. Salt and season to taste and cook for another hour.

OMG SMOOTHIE

In your blender, drop a handful of frozen banana chunks, 1 cup soy

or almond milk, 1/2 cup or so frozen berries. Whir the heck out of it.

Pour into a tall glass. It is too good to be true.

COOKING GRAINS
(like quinoa, bulgur and brown rice, or lentils)

If you have a rice cooker, use that. Rinse lentils or grains first, then use proportions of 1 to 2: i.e., 1 cup lentils or grain to 2 cups water, 2 cups lentils or grain to 4 cups water, etc. Okay to salt before cooking. On the stove: same proportions. Put grains or legumes into large saucepan. Add twice the amount of water. Salt (always optional but I can't live without it.) Bring to a boil, then turn down to lowest simmer and cover. Cook for 15 minutes. Turn off heat. Leave cover on. Let sit another 5 minutes or until all water is absorbed. Fluff with fork and serve as stir fry base, add a handful to your soup, stuff a whole-grain burrito with this plus some salsa, cook up a mess of kale and toss in a cup of cooked grains.
NOTE: wheat berries don't cook like grains. They cook more like beans, meaning you have to cook the heck out of them before they soften.

GAS FREE BEANS

In a big saucepan with a lid, pour in 1 pound of dry beans (or one bag) and wash well under running water. Drain. Add enough water to cover plus another 3 inches or so. (Doesn't really matter.) On high heat, bring the beans and water to a boil. Boil hard for 3 minutes. Turn heat off. Cover the pan and let it sit for 30 minutes or so. Drain all the water off. Run more water over the beans until all bubbles are gone. Add water to cover again plus 2 inches, add 1-2 T. olive oil, and bring to a boil.

Crock pot: As soon as the water has boiled the second time, dump it all into your crock pot, and cook the beans on low for 8 hours or high for 4 hours.) Add salt at the end.

Stovetop: When the water boils, reduce the heat to as low as possible but still bubbling (simmering) cover with lid and cook for an hour or more. The beans need to be WELL cooked. This is key to the gas-free part. Some of them will be broken, falling apart. If in doubt, cook longer. Add salt ONLY at the end.

COOKING GREENS

(like collards and kale)

Remove twist tie and wash greens thoroughly. One leaf at a time, fold in half lengthwise and slice off the thick stem. Discard. Take the remaining leaves and chop in thin horizontal strips, about 1/2 inch wide. In wok or other frying pan, heat 1 T. olive oil. Toss in 1-3 cloves chopped garlic, and immediately toss in the greens. They may overflow the pan at first, but they will wilt down as you heat and turn them. They will be finished in 5 minutes. Add salt, hot sauce, vinegar or lemon juice, soy sauce - whatever you like. Delicious and beautiful served atop beans and/or grains.

ROASTING ROOT VEGETABLES

(like turnips, rutabaga, parsnips, carrots)

Cut up big mouthsized chunks of your favorite root vegetables, plus onions and potatoes if you like. In a big flat oven-proof pan, toss all the veggies with just a bit of olive oil, plus salt and pepper and your favorite dry herbs. Bake in 400 degree oven for about 30 minutes. (Check after 15 minutes to see if potatoes are done. If they're done, the rest is done, too.) Serve hot.

ROASTING OTHER VEGETABLES

(like Brussels sprouts, green beans, asparagus, peppers, broccoli, cauliflower...anything you can think of, except maybe peas)

Cut into bite-sized chunks, coat with olive oil, salt and seasonings,

and roast in a very hot oven (500 degrees) for about 10 minutes.

Yum.

Of course, you can add the second group of vegetables to the pan of

root vegetables after the root vegetables have cooked for 15 minutes

or so. You'll figure this out. Ovens vary, and this method is very

forgiving.

Save leftovers to eat as a snack, or add to soup, or mix up with your

greens and grains, roll up in a tortilla, or or or...

Works Cited

Avena, Maddy. Weblog post. BodyTales. <Bodytales.blogspot.com>.

CattleNetwork - Cattle Beef Homepage. 01 Oct. 2008
        <http://Cattlenetwork.com>.

Free Diet Plans at SparkPeople. 1 Oct. 2008 <http://sparkpeople.com>.

Free Healthy Recipes! Nutrition, Weight Loss Topics And Free Cook
        Books. 1 Oct. 2008 <http://healthrecipes.com>.

GoVeg.com: Vegetarian and Vegan Information. 1 Oct. 2008
        <http://goveg.com>.

The Harvard Medical School Guide to Healthy Eating. New York: Simon
        and Schuster, 2001.

Harvard School of Public Health - HSPH. 1 Oct. 2008
        <http://www.hsph.harvard.edu>.

Journal of Animal Science. 1 Oct. 2008 <http://jas.fass.org>.

Middle Eastern Food at About.com - Middle Eastern Food Recipes. 01
        Oct. 2008 <http://mideastfood.about.com>.

My Jewish Learning - Exploring Judaism & Jewish Life. 1 Oct. 2008
        <http://myjewishlearning.com>.

Nestle, Marion. Food Politics: How the Food Industry Influences Nutrition
        and Health. University of California, 2003.

Oklahoma Cooperative Extension Service. 1 Oct. 2008
        <http://osufacts.okstate.edu>.

Polakow, Melody. Weblog post. Melomeals. <melomeals.blogspot.com>.

Schlosser, Eric. Fast Food Nation - The Dark Side of the All-American
        Meal. New York: Houghton-Mifflin, 2001.

U.S. USDA. Nutritive Value of American Foods in Common Units -
        Handbook. Vol. 456.

Vegetarian Recipes | VegCooking.com.
      <http://vegcooking.com>.